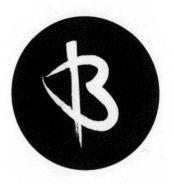

BROTHERS

Brothers

Every man needs strong, authentic friendships

Kim Evensen

Cover photo: Susan L'Estrange Photography

ISBN-13: 978-0-6484829-0-1

I know that this book will impact friendships all over the world…

I'm proud of you.

Love,

Your friend and brother

Vaughn

BROTHERS

CONTENTS

Foreword   v

1   The beginning   1

2   The importance of male friendship   7

3   Growing up as a sensitive boy   11

4   I love you bro (no homo)   19

5   Help, I'm a man and I need comfort!   25

6   Let's talk about manhood   31

7   Superman is desperate for friendship   37

8   Often believed myths about men and men's   39
    friendships

9   A world obsessed with romantic love   47

10 What is a friendship built on?   53

11 An organisation about men's friendships.   63
    Sounds a bit awkward, doesn't it?

12 You're not the only one   67

13 Meet Ayden, my new best friend   69

14 Sidenote   77

15 Comparison and competition   79

16 See you later, bro   85

17 When the rubber hits the road   89

18 Friends for a season or friends for life?   91

19 Don't ditch your bro for a woman   93

20 Why veterans miss war   99

21 When it doesn't go as planned   103

22 Brother, I'm coming back!   109

23 It's normal   117

24 Practical advice   123

25 The journey ahead   133

26 Join the journey   139

ACKNOWLEDGMENTS

First, this book is for all my boys who I'm privileged to live life with.

Thanks to Colin Emerson for encouraging me and helping me write this book, Susan L'Estrange for the cover photo, and thanks to Amanda Clark (Brothers' co-leader) and all our volunteers for fighting alongside me. Thanks to Niobe Way, Mark Greene and Judy Y Chu for your encouragement, advice and wisdom. You've prepared the way for Brothers.

ABOUT THE AUTHOR

Kim Evensen, twenty-six, is the CEO and founder of
Brothers. He was born in Norway but lives in
Australia. He has three years of leadership education,
four years of acting education, and he studies men's
development and friendships independently.

ABOUT BROTHERS

Brothers is a global movement that seeks to empower and inspire boys and men to create strong, wholesome and authentic friendships and combat damaging cultural influences that can hinder this. We aim to change men's lives and pioneer growth in male friendships.

www.wearebrothers.org

DISCLAIMER

The names of some people in this book have been changed to protect their privacy.

This book is about Kim's journey of friendship. Kim is not responsible for any actions you may take, or others' reactions, when applying what you learn from this book to your own life. Kim is not a professional psychologist or counsellor, and he does not provide professional mental health advice or support.

FOREWORD
By Mark Greene

In November of 2017, Kim Evensen Skyped me from Norway. He had founded *Brothers*. He already had some pretty impressive branding and a classy logo. The project had the polish and appeal of a fashion shoot. There were photographs of young men arm in arm. *Brothers'* mission was to encourage young men's friendships.

I remember thinking, "Okay. Um... Cool."

The irony of my initial response is not lost on me. I had been writing for years about the brutal mechanisms by which our dominant culture of manhood strips boys of their natural capacity to form meaningful, authentic friendships. As a result, millions of men are facing a deadly epidemic of loneliness. This is literally at the core of my work and I'm like, "Yeah. Okay. Sure, why not?"

I attribute my response to the following. On some level, when I saw *Brothers'* pictures of young men connecting, I couldn't quite relate, because like many of us, I don't really know how to process images of close male friendships, having seen so very few of them in my own life.

Western culture is collectively transfixed by images of the angry men who have come to define our society's most damaging narratives about manhood. This rage, all our collective social, political and cultural challenges comes down to one thing.

Millions of us, boys and men alike, are infected with a deep-seated and alienating loneliness. This loneliness is at the heart of every dysfunction that plagues us. It is a loneliness created by a culture of manhood that from earliest childhood shames and bullies us away from wanting and needing genuine, heartfelt friendships.

Which is why *Brothers*' mission is so powerful. Along comes *Brothers* saying, "Hey guys. Here's what real friendship can look like," presenting images and stories born of Kim Evensen's own deep need for connection.

Kim knows the work of the leaders in the field. He understands exactly how our culture of manhood goes about brutally shaming and isolating generations of men. He could be focusing on telling that story, but by filling social media with rich, compelling images and messages about the power and grace of young men's friendships, *Brothers* is instead creating something entirely radical: permission.

Brothers' work grants us permission to love our friends, revealing, in turn, the deepest most surprising truth of male friendship: that we can love each other with such compassion that it will fuel a lifetime of vibrant connection, no matter our age, race, class, orientation or history.

And these are the friendships that will heal the world.

Mark Greene
Author, *The Little #MeToo Book for Men*

BROTHERS

1 THE BEGINNING

I'm writing this book because I hope it will make a
difference to people's lives, especially men's. I want to
see boys and men across the world develop authentic,
wholesome and purposeful friendships. I believe none
of us have been created to live mediocre lives, so we
shouldn't settle for mediocre friendships.

Some guys might find my message confronting.
You might realise that the friendships you've got aren't
as deep as you thought they were. That might be a
painful realisation, but trust me, it's an important one.
The first step is to see what needs to change. Some
guys might be inspired to fight for a friendship they've
let fade away. Others might feel disconnected in their
current friendships. You might feel like your
friendships are empty or lack depth. Maybe you're one
of many who've settled for mediocre friendships,

believing that's all there is, and you might not even be keen on anything deeper. If that's you, this book may change your mind. Others may have given up on friendships altogether due to betrayal or life's seasons and challenges. You might not even want friendships in your life anymore. I hope this book will make you believe in friendship again.

I've encountered countless guys who simply think they've got it all sorted out and don't get the point of Brothers. But if you have a wife or a girlfriend – do you think the attitude 'I'm a perfect husband so I don't need to work on it' would be good for your relationship? That would be naive, irresponsible and destructive. So why do we treat our friendships differently?

For our friendships to grow, we must admit they're not perfect. If we think our friendships don't need any work or 'maintenance', we're fooling ourselves. If we think we 'know it all' when it comes to friendships, we've just revealed that we don't. My advice when reading this book is for you to have an open and receptive heart. Follow that advice, and this book might just change your life.

Many men will find it weird to read a book on men's friendships, let alone just *talk* about them. You might think that it sounds 'super gay' – and the fact that you've started reading this book is a miracle in itself. You might be totally satisfied with the casual hang-outs with the boys in your life. A beer at a bar, chatting about sports and women – that's what you want, and you're not keen on anything deeper. Well, I'm stoked that you've picked up this book, and I encourage you to finish it. Who knows ... Maybe this book will alter your perception of friendship for the better. There's only one way to find out.

A few days ago, I had a chat with Niobe Way. She's a professor of developmental psychology at New York University and the author of multiple books and hundreds of journal articles, and most importantly, she's been researching friendships among boys for years. She's someone I respect, and I thank her for her research, wisdom and insight into male relationships. Anyway, as we were chatting about boys and friendship over the phone, she talked about the importance of normalising boys' and men's desire and longing for friendship in a culture that doesn't allow them to. Popular culture might say that boys and men don't need or want friendship – they are hardwired to just want casual hang-outs – but research and my experience as the founder of Brothers shows something different. Niobe's research with teenage boys indicates that about 80% of them speak openly in their interviews about their deep affection and love for their best male friends. They even express deep sadness if in a conflict with a friend. She also told me about an occasion when she was discussing friendships with a classroom of twelve-year-old boys. After she read aloud a passage from her book (where one of the interviewed boys talks explicitly about his deep affection for his best friend), the boys in the classroom started giggling. Niobe knew exactly why, but she still asked why they were laughing. At first, none of the boys wanted to tell her, but after a little while, one of the boys said, 'Well … because he sounds gay.'

Of course, Niobe knew what the boys would answer, but she wanted them to put words to it themselves. And she took the chance to remind them that desiring close friendship – and even being hurt when facing trials in our friendships – is normal and good, and that it has nothing to do with our sexuality but all to do with our humanity. She told them that most teenage boys sound like this over the course of adolescence. There was silence in the room. And then boys started opening up about their longing for deep friendships.

What Niobe did here was normalise the boys' desire for connections with other boys. These boys had different personalities, but they all had this in common. So whatever kind of guy you are – if you're an emotional dude or not very emotional at all – you need friendship. Despite your nationality, age, race, class or sphere of life, you were created for it. My goal with this book is to share with you my journey of friendship, my struggles with it and my need for it, and hopefully empower you and your friendships as well.

But hey, let me give you a little bit of an introduction. My name is Kim Evensen. I'm a twenty-six-year-old guy from Norway, but I currently live in Australia. As mentioned, I'm the founder of an organisation called Brothers, and the best introduction to Brothers is our mission statement:

> Brothers is a global movement that seeks to empower and inspire boys and men to create strong, wholesome and authentic friendships, and combat damaging cultural influences that can hinder this.

So yeah, an organisation about men's friendships. In this book you'll read more about my journey, Brothers, and why I started Brothers in the first place. I'll write about my own experiences with friendship (as a boy and as a man), and how I've dealt with closeness, authenticity and vulnerability in my male relationships.

My goal is that, as you read the book, you'll be informed, inspired and provoked to thought. I hope you recognise yourself in my story. I know we're all different, but we've got so much in common. And even though this book is written mainly for men, I hope that it'll inspire women to invest in their friendships and encourage the men in their lives to do the same. Strong friendships in your man's life will benefit not only him but also all his relationships – yes, our whole society.

2 THE IMPORTANCE OF MALE FRIENDSHIP

I'm glad there are more and more organisations out there focusing on men's health, but most of these organisations have forgotten about *friendship*. They talk about marriage, kids, work, sex, physical, emotional and mental health – but they have little or no information about friendship, though the consequences of the lack of deep male bonding in a man's life[1] are many:

- greater risk of social isolation (which can lead to stress-related illness, isolation, addiction, suicide, divorce, violence, abuse and crime)

---

[1] N Way, *Deep Secrets: Boys' Friendships and the Crisis of Connection*, Harvard University Press, Cambridge MA, 2011; JY Chu, *When Boys Become Boys: Development, Relationships, and Masculinity*, NYU Press, New York, 2014; R Garfield, *Breaking The Male* Code, Avery, New York, 2016.

- decreased lifespan (more likelihood of Alzheimer's, heart disease, obesity, diabetes, high blood pressure, neurodegenerative diseases and even cancer)

- less productivity in one's personal and professional life

- lack of resources and resiliency in times of crisis

- poorer connection with spouse, kids, peers, family and themselves.

Niobe Way says that

> when adolescent boys stop sharing their intimate feelings with their peers, we see an alarming increase in their rates of depression and suicide. Wives who cite their husband's 'emotional unavailability' as the primary cause of divorce initiate two out of every three divorces today.[2]

In the newly published book *The Crisis of Connection: Roots, Consequences and Solutions* by Niobe Way, Alisha Ali, Carol Gilligan and Pedro Noguera, we read that the absence of close friendships also negatively affects

---

[2] R Garfield, *Breaking The Male* Code, Avery, New York, 2016.

a person's physical health and lower one's resistance to illness.[3]

So we're not fighting for men's friendships because we think it's a cool thing to do. We fight for these vital relationships in a man's life because it changes lives and societies alike.

---

[3] Way, N., Ali, A., Gilligan, C., Noguera, P. and Kirkland, D. (2018). *The crisis of connection.* 1st ed. NYU Press.

BROTHERS

3 GROWING UP AS A SENSITIVE BOY

I grew up in a small town in Norway, about one and a half hours from Oslo. I was a joyful and happy boy who would connect with people easily, no matter what age they were. I remember I met an elderly woman when I was about eight or nine years old (while on vacation with my family), and we ended up becoming best friends. Almost every day after school, I'd go straight to her flat and cook for her and eat with her. Fried eggs and potatoes. We'd have long conversations about life and just enjoy each other's company. One day, after arriving home from a holiday, my parents sat down with me to have a chat. They told me that my best friend had died while I was away.

***

At school I was the good boy. I did very well, and I often did more homework than I had to. (I loved getting credit and encouragements from the teachers.) I was sensitive, caring and interested in people. I tried joining the soccer team when I was six but realised it wasn't my thing. I was afraid of the ball. So I joined the church choir instead – I found that much more fun.

In the beginning it didn't bother the other boys in my class that I didn't like sport – we still connected. I loved playing with Lego and running around in the forest and building tree houses. But as we grew older it changed. Being a boy meant that you'd have to behave in a certain way or face the consequences.

I was eight years old, and most of the boys started toughening up – almost as a way of surviving. I, on the other hand, just kept displaying my feelings. On top of that, I was a Christian. So you can do the math … A sensitive, openminded Christian boy (who didn't like sports but liked singing and dancing). I became the most popular boy, and the lads thought I was rad. Not.

I ended up more or less being rejected by the boys. The girls, on the other hand, embraced me. They were loving and caring. They would listen to me. They wouldn't push me away if I expressed my emotions. They loved me. The boys wouldn't really relate to me because I hung out with girls and didn't like the things 'a boy was expected to like' or behaved in the way 'a boy was expected to behave'.

I had a group of girl friends I got really close to. Among them was a girl named Leah. We used to hang out every day at school – and often after school. She ended up becoming my first girlfriend, and we dated for almost one and a half years. So here I was, ten years old, with lots of girl friends – and a girlfriend – but I simply didn't fit in among the boys, though I really wanted to.

Fast forward a few years. I was in junior high and officially a teenager at thirteen years old. The guys had become even more tough, emotionally stoic, and they avoided closeness in their friendships at all costs. The only closeness a guy could be interested in was with a girl. Sexual closeness, really. But I still kept revealing my emotions. I didn't want to sleep around. And I desired authentic friendships with people. The consequences were no guy friendships, no 'being one of the boys', and I'd be called gay, a wuss and a girl until I got used to it.

There was a lot of turbulence in my family in my teenage years. That, plus the bullying and rejection I faced daily in school, affected me more than I was aware. I remember I went to counselling once or twice a week to talk about life. I think I cried every session. Oh, goodness … The sensitive boy. Gotta love it. Anyway, I remember this new dude who started at my school, having moved to our town from another. He was really cool, and I enjoyed our conversations. He was genuine. I was fifteen years old at this point, and it was a perfect opportunity for me to finally build a friendship with another *guy* – but I had to hurry up before the other boys in school would screw it up for me. Unfortunately, it didn't take long until the other boys told this guy, 'Kim's a girl, a nerd, gay, a Christian' (which wasn't considered as very cool), etc. So he ended up following their advice (I don't blame him) and staying away from me. The cost was too high for him to pay.

One day when I was chatting with my counsellor about the new guy, I told her about everything. I expressed great sadness because he didn't want to be my friend (after what the other boys had told him). After I had gotten it all off my chest, I remember my counsellor paused and asked me, 'Kim, have you ever considered that you might be gay?' For a moment I thought she was joking. I couldn't really take her seriously. Did she ask if I was gay? I talked about *friendship* – what's gay about that? Realising she wasn't joking, I looked at her and said no, but she still really doubted my answer. The rest of our conversation was mostly about her trying to convince me that I was gay – and it pissed me off. I trusted her, and I opened up to her – but apparently, as a guy, I wasn't supposed to have those needs. It took me years to realise that what I felt wasn't unnatural, unmanly or weird. I was human, and I realise now that what I did was bold. I refused to conform to toxic, stereotypical gender norms. I wanted to keep my humanity.

(Keep in mind that I respect all people regardless of their sexual preference. I'm just challenging our culture's sexualisation of love and friendship.)

My counsellor never meant to be mean, but she revealed that she had a very limited perception of masculinity and male bonding. And she's not the only one. I've encountered countless teachers, leaders and mentors who've got the exact same issue. They quickly label boys' natural behaviour (sensitivity, desire for friendship, warmth and joy) as gay or girlish. This is limiting and destructive to them, to their relationships and to our whole society. And if our teachers and role models have this mindset, new generations will too.

Looking back, I understand why I went through all this. I needed this experience to be able to run Brothers – and to help guys develop worthwhile friendships in their own lives. But at the time, it wasn't cool, and it led to me being rejected because I wanted real friendship, because I didn't want to put on a tough, 'masculine' mask. Part of me started to believe that guys simply shouldn't want or need close, warm friendships.

A few years later I started high school. I was keen on acting and theatre, so I studied that. There were *three* boys in our class – and twenty-seven girls. As I've said, I was used to being friends with girls, so it wasn't new to me. But since I really wanted to identify with the boys, I did everything I could to avoid being friends with girls. I hadn't really felt like one of the guys before, and I wanted to change that.

I still remember one hang-out with this guy called Andy. We'd met at school but started hanging out outside of school too. I was sixteen, and it was a few days before Christmas Eve. We went to his place, and I got to meet his mum as well. I stayed over that night, and after we had pulled out the extra mattress for me to sleep on, brushed our teeth and gotten into bed, we started *talking* – like when you're both really tired and you start talking about the *deep stuff* – and I remember I was *stoked* about it. I thought to myself,

I'm actually getting a bro! Oh, yeah! And we're having a sleep-over. This is just sick. I'm one of the boys now! I had waited for years to connect with other guys. Finally, it happened.

BROTHERS

4 I LOVE YOU, BRO (NO HOMO)

As a guy, have you ever avoided closeness (either emotional or physical) in any of your friendships with guys? Have you ever added a 'no homo' after expressing some form of affection or appreciation towards a guy friend?

A few years ago, I moved to Australia to study. Long story short, I ended up meeting a dude called Ayden, who later became my closest friend. And my experiences in that friendship are a big part of why I started Brothers.

I'm not afraid of expressing affection. To this day, people think of me as a 'ball of joy'. Just like a three-year-old boy, I express love and affection towards the people I love with no shame. It's beautiful. But it costs.

I remember I wanted to post a photo of me and Ayden on Facebook. You know, just another selfie with my bro. Anyway, I started writing some nice stuff about him in the caption, and when I showed it to him before posting it, he got a bit awkward and suggested that I might make it a bit less affectionate. A bit less loving. I remember I asked why, and he said that 'people might get the wrong idea'. I knew exactly what he meant. And it annoyed the heck out of me. But I ended up writing something like, 'This is my brother from another mother! Really appreciate you, man!' when I actually wanted to write, 'I love this guy *so* much.'

Ayden and I went to the gym one day, and this woman we'd met a few times before was in the sauna. As we chatted, she suddenly asked us, 'So when are you going to take your relationship to the next level?' She had a cheeky smile. I didn't know what to say, but Ayden just brushed it off and started talking about something else. When we got out of the sauna and were on our way home, Ayden could see that I was thinking a lot. He asked if I was still thinking about what that woman said. I was. And I was pissed off. 'How dare she?! As if our friendship isn't good

enough without it being sexual. That's just stupid.'
Ayden told me to not worry about it.

Another time, I was hugging one of my closest
friends (after hanging out) and some guys were driving
by and shouting 'gay!' out the window. Multiple times
I've been frowned upon when expressing love towards
a guy friend – people laughing and saying 'that's gay' as
they continue talking about something else.

Okay. So what's the problem here?

Well, the problem is the sexualisation of love.
Consider this: we are constantly being bombarded
with sexual messages. Music, movies, ads – you name
it. And it affects the way we look at life, at love, at
relationships. I like to ask guys what comes to their
minds when I say words like 'intimacy' or 'closeness'
or 'love'. Most of the time, they think sex. No wonder
many male friendships lack intimacy! Our culture has
reserved intimacy for sexual relationships only.

Let's picture a little boy. Do you think he's afraid
of expressing *gentle* emotional or physical affection
towards his best guy friend? Well, probably not. He
wouldn't even think about it. If he likes someone, he'll
gladly express it. But imagine a twenty-year-old guy.
Do you think he might find it challenging to express
this kind of love towards his buddy? I do – I've found
it challenging myself. Both to express and to receive

such love from another guy. That I find it challenging reveals there's something really wrong going on – and it ought to be dealt with.

It's okay to be close to another guy when you're three years old. But not when you're older. Because that's gay. Apparently. But if you're a woman, it's much more accepted. Picture two women looking into each other's eyes, smiling and giving each other a warm hug. Would you assume that their relationship would be sexual? Now picture two guys doing the same. What would you assume?

'Well, Kim. This just sounds like a cuddle club. And honestly, guys simply don't need close guy friendships. Guys just hang out. That's what they do. Shoulder-to-shoulder friendships. Not the whole face-to-face thing. Women do that. Not guys.'

My mission is not to turn men's friendships into a cuddle club – we all express love in different ways. But if we think that closeness is only reserved for dating relationships, we're doing ourselves a huge disfavour.

I once chatted to this guy about closeness and comfort. He said that he really wanted closeness, but he didn't have a girlfriend. I asked him, 'Well, can't you get this closeness from your guy friends?' He didn't think so.

Last question: have you ever wondered why it's fine for male athletes to hug and be physical during a football match but not for average guy on the street? Here's my answer: they're 'allowed' to express themselves like this because they're *already doing* something that is considered *masculine*. So they know they can hug, kiss or slap a teammate's bum after scoring a goal without their masculinity or heterosexuality being questioned. Being an athlete (doing something 'masculine') works as a cover for them to express themselves in ways that otherwise would've labelled them gay.

BROTHERS

5 HELP, I'M A MAN AND I NEED COMFORT!

(A PREVIOUSLY PUBLISHED ARTICLE)

I love that Brothers has 'forced me' to be more open about things. If I'm going to lead a movement of men desiring deeper friendships, I need to be bold and sometimes choose the way less travelled, ask uncomfortable questions, open up about things others wouldn't open up about – you get it.

Softness, vulnerability and emotionality are at the core of our humanity, says Niobe Way. Both young girls and boys desire and need safety and closeness. It's not something we learn; it's something we are born with. And babies and children are pretty good at expressing their need for it. But we all know that if you don't practise a skill, you may lose it. So it is with our ability to give and receive comfort. Parents love to see their little boys connect with others – and it's beautiful to see them generously give and receive affection. But somewhere along the way, boys are taught not to do this. As Mark Greene puts it, they are actually trained away from it.

I find it so much easier to open up to girls or women about my struggles. Even though I do have male friends, yes, even a best guy friend, I find it difficult to go to him when I need any form of compassion. And honestly, it hurts to admit that. I do want to receive comfort from him. I do want to be able to sit next to a brother and even lean on his shoulder and know that it's okay to do so. But I often don't ask. I've burned myself before, so I'd rather play it safe and be quiet about it. I know that just seeking help elsewhere is easier than opening my heart to a 'best friend' and being rejected. I would rather believe that the friendship is perfect and not ask for comfort, because I know that asking for it might reveal that the friendship isn't as solid as I imagined.

I said to a woman the other day, 'You know, sometimes I hate being a boy.' (I normally don't use the word 'hate' like that, because it's a strong word … But I guess after so much frustration, I just needed to use that word to describe how I've felt over a long period of time.) I told her that, as a man, it is so difficult to get solace from my friends. We laughed, but she admitted that she had thought this herself, and she was glad she was a woman when it came to this. I continued to open up to her. The feeling of being rejected when seeking help from someone you call your best friend is heartbreaking. We had a long and serious conversation about this, but we also laughed about the whole thing as well; it's kind of a tragicomedy.

Anyway, seeking any form of comfort from a guy is for me often very difficult. But then there's also the rejection when *giving* it. And please know that there are times when we just don't want it, when we need space. And let us be gracious and respect one another for that. But I am talking about all those times I have tried to extend help to a brother but he has been unable to receive it. Why? Well. Many men simply don't believe that they're supposed to give or receive any form of comfort – and especially not from other men. So when they receive solace from another man, an alarm bell goes off, shouting, 'This is not normal. This is weird. This is no good. I don't need this.'

Knowing this has helped me be patient when experiencing rejection by close male friends. Even though I have sometimes left feeling stupid and humiliated, I need to remind myself of this one belief I want to live by: 'Just continue to love them.' Because that's what I want them to do to me.

But I wonder where many men turn to for compassion, since many of them don't get it from their friends. I wonder how many men go to the club to get 'closeness'. They find a woman (or a guy for that matter), they hook up and end up in bed – and their desire for genuine connection conflates with their sexual desires, leading to a false comfort. I believe that if a man doesn't have a place to be warmly welcomed and embraced, he will get something 'like it' somewhere else, whether it's sex, porn, drugs, alcohol – even career or fitness, for that matter.

And to all the married men out there: I do hope you receive closeness and support from not only your wife but also from your mates. If you're relying *only* on her for closeness, you're placing a burden on her that she should not and cannot carry alone. So do her and yourself a favour, and make sure you have a friendship that allows you to find comfort and closeness.

You might recognise yourself in some of this chapter. I hope you did. If so, my message is this: men, don't shy away from receiving or giving comfort, whether physical (affection) or with words (affirmation). You were created for it, and the sooner you realise that, the better. Those moments when you shy away from it, think about your brother, think about your friend. A hug from you, a shoulder from you, might mean the world to him. He might not dare to admit that it does, but that's okay. Dare to give and receive comfort, even if you know you might face rejection.

6 LET'S TALK ABOUT MANHOOD

When I became a teenager, I started being extra aware of how I acted, the way I talked. I remember trying not to cross my legs when sitting, because that felt a little 'girlish'. I also had a period when I was extremely conscious of how I walked. I would look at myself in the mirror when walking towards it, making sure I walked in a 'masculine' way. All because I didn't want anyone to think that I was less of a man, gay or girlish.

I wonder how much time we as men in western culture spend (either consciously or unconsciously) on proving our manhood or heterosexuality. We carefully choose our words and actions, making sure that we express *nothing* other than manliness.

In *Breaking the Male Code*, Dr Robert Garfield writes about a set of behaviours that many men subscribe to. Though this 'code' isn't very much spoken about, it has a lot of power in the lives of men. The 'code' sounds like this:

- Don't express your emotions (other than anger, 'manly' emotions or excitement over sports).

- Be tough, rough and strong.

- Don't express too much joy or admiration when hanging out with the boys. (This might be suspicious.)

- Remember to talk about sport and 'masculine' activities to reaffirm to yourself and the guys that you're a *man*.

- Be a womaniser – because *real men* can score whenever they want to.

- Be independent and in control.

And by all means, avoid expressing any of these things:

- sensitivity and warm emotions

- dependence on others

- loss of control

- any expression that could be considered feminine or gay.

As men go about our lives, we're under constant scrutiny by other men: Follow the code. Don't do anything that makes other men suspicious of your masculinity or heterosexuality. And if you break this code, be ready for disaster. It can result in total abandonment by other men. And who wants that? I certainly don't. I want the guys in my life to respect me, to admire me and to think that I'm a man. So I better just follow the 'code' then ...

Doesn't this sound exhausting? Well, many men are pretty good at playing this game. It has become second nature, the normal way of behaving. But though following the 'male code' will give you acceptance from other men, it'll have serious consequences for your family, marriage, relationships and society. No wonder so many women complain about their man's emotional unavailability. He's bound to the 'male code'. He's been told since the day he was born that men shouldn't feel or express warmth, love or dependence on other people. As a child, the little boy appreciated warmth, love and gentleness, but as he grew up, he was shamed away from it, feeling that it's 'wrong' for him to feel or express these emotions. In Niobe Way's book *Deep Secrets*, we follow a few guys as they enter adolescence. When I read Way's book, I observed that these guys get stuck in this *limbo*. One part of them wants and desires close, intimate friendships with their peers, but another part of them feels like they shouldn't want, desire or need that – because that's not manly. It was okay when they were kids, but not as *men*. Therefore, as these guys grew up, they started trading away their emotional sensitivity to be 'one of the boys'. By doing that they actually lost their ability to form worthwhile relationships. By trying to fit in, they missed out.

I've experienced this limbo myself, and I still am, to an extent. But I've promised myself that I will continue to fight against the 'male code'. I deserve better. And so do the people in my life.

I have often asked women if they feel like they need to 'prove their womanhood'. Most of the time I get a no. But when asking guys if they've ever felt like they need to prove their manhood, I mostly get a yes. I find that very interesting. Growing up, I've heard the phrase 'man up' many times (and I haven't really reflected on why; I've just accepted it.) When I've wanted to cry, I've been told to get over it. When I've wanted closeness or comfort, I've been told to get laid or get a girlfriend. When I've wanted closer connections with guys, I've received disapproval.

As a man, I've been exposed to so many messages on 'how to be man enough' – and they've all left me feeling like a failure. I've realised that I'm not measuring up to those standards of manhood, no matter how hard I try. An attendee at a Brothers event put it like this: 'The cultural expectations of a man are impossible to reach. If you try to reach them, you'll always find yourself falling short.'

Not only are you reaching for something impossible to reach, you're also trying to attain something that is damaging to you and those around you. If you really want to be tough, in control, independent and emotionally stoic, then go for it. It's your life. But you'll miss out on the depth of real friendship and connection with people.

This is what I tell guys who ask me questions about 'being man enough': *You don't need to prove anything.* You don't need to prove to other men, to your wife, to your children or anyone that you're a man. You simply are.

7 SUPERMAN IS DESPERATE FOR FRIENDSHIP

The culture we live in affects the way we behave. And if we're not aware of this, we can end up in great danger.

Think about all the entertainment we consume daily: TV shows, movies, music, ads – you name it. Take movies; describe the main male characters in most action and superhero movies. How do they behave, and what do they want? Do they have any close friendships? Are they loving or caring towards others, or do they appear strong, emotionally stoic and independent? Last time I watched a Superman movie, he wasn't really into friendships. He was a lone, strong wolf, trying to save the world and win the girl.

I do like these kinds of movies; they're cool. A part of me would love to identify with the heroes in the movies; they make me feel like ... a man. And I want to feel like a man, don't I? But let's be real. If I'd become friends with Superman, I don't think we'd have the best or the deepest friendship – it would take time for him to relearn how to be close to people. Superman might be cool, but he's not a good role model when it comes to building worthwhile relationships.

What about other movies, such as comedies? In most comedies I've watched, the main character's friends are mostly stupid, lazy or there to encourage him to get laid. Sometimes the male protagonist might have a friendship, but it's often just a series of shallow hang-outs.

So here's my point: if we let popular culture set the standards for our friendships, we won't attain many meaningful ones. I don't want friendships that look like those portrayed in popular media.

Question: When was the last time you saw a loving friendship between two guys in a movie?

8 OFTEN BELIEVED MYTHS ABOUT MEN AND MEN'S FRIENDSHIPS

Here are some commonly believed myths about men and men's friendships:

- Men are not interested in close friendships with other men.

- Men aren't wired to be emotionally intimate with other people.

- Men are only interested in sex.

- Men's friendships are more like 'shoulder to shoulder' but women's friendships are more like 'face to face'.

- Men's friendships are about what we *do* together; women's friendships are about *being* together.

You might think some of those myths aren't myths at all. If that's you, I'd ask you to keep an open mind as we continue. To begin with I want to suggest that emotional awareness and the desire for close friendships is a *human* quality, not a feminine one.

Before moving forward, I'd like to discuss a few common assertions about men's friendships:

'Me and my best bro only catch up every now and then. But when we catch up, it's like nothing has changed. We don't need to hang out a lot, but we're still super close.'

My response to that is:

Me: So, do you love your brother?

Him: Yeah.

Me: Do you believe that you make a difference in each other's lives?

Him: Definitely.

Me: But you don't you spend a lot of time with him, right?

Him: No, but we're still close.

Me: Okay. Cool. Have you ever had a girlfriend?

Him: Yeah.

Me: Did you spend a lot of time with her?

Him: Of course I did.

Me: Why's that?

Him: Well, we loved each other. And we loved being with each other, and for our relationship to grow we needed to spend time together.

Me: Too easy. What if you had a kid? Would you spend time with him?

Him: Of course. Anything else would be silly.

Me: Then why do you treat your friendships differently?

Him: …

A lot of guys might say, 'But you can't compare a girlfriend with a best friend.'

But says who? Of course I can. And the fact that many guys respond like that shows that they've deprioritised friendships to something that doesn't need investment or care – and why is that? Well, CS Lewis suggests in his book *The Four Loves* that many don't value friendship because they haven't *experienced* real friendship. You simply can't have a close, growing relationship with *anyone* without spending time together. You can't enjoy the ongoing depth and closeness of a relationship without commitment.

Here's another observation I've made. You might have heard about this popular meme about male vs female friendships:

> Guy friendships:
>
> Guy 1: Dude, you're an arsehole.
>
> Guy 2: Thanks, man. You're a bigger one.
>
> *They laugh together and their friendship lasts for life.*
>
> Women's friendships:
>
> Woman 1: Girl, I love you so much! You mean so much to me.
>
> Woman 2: I love you too! I don't know where I would've been without you.
>
> *They look into each other's eyes and hug each other. Their friendship lasts for six months.*

Reading this you might think 'that's so true!' but I don't think either of these caricatures are very helpful.

I believe one of the reasons some of these (not very encouraging) male friendships last a lifetime is that they're not *deep* enough. So whenever their friend does something that normally (in a deep friendship) would've hurt them, they don't care – and they won't confront their friend about it. Why? Because there's no emotional intimacy in their friendship. No depth, no turbulence. No turbulence, and a friendship might last a lifetime (just like a car that never gets driven).

In a lot of female friendships, emotional intimacy and expression is accepted and even encouraged. That's a good thing, but again, that doesn't mean that their friendships are necessarily deep. Words are cheap if our actions don't back them up. If we say, 'I love you,' we should also *show it*. I've encountered women showering their girlfriends with words of affirmation they don't really mean. If that's the case, then yes – I understand why their friendship might last for only six months.

I've seen both women's *and* men's friendships last 'forever', and I've also seen both last for a short season only. And there might be many reasons that determine a friendship's length. But I believe that if a friendship is deep enough, it will endure *turbulence*. What we do when we face conflicts is up to us. Do we fight for each other or do we flee from each other?

I also want to highlight the importance of speaking positively and using our words to build each other up. There's nothing I love more than hearing a brother tell me how much he loves me. But again, words are dead without action. You can't say you love someone without showing them. But it's also important to tell people that you love them as well. If you find it difficult to do this, then start practising. A clumsy and stuttering 'I really care about you' is all it takes.

My wish is for you to have both long-lasting *and* deep friendships. But remember that long-lasting friendships aren't necessarily healthy ones.

Shoulder-to-shoulder friendships

It sounds so nice: 'Men's friendships are more like shoulder-to-shoulder friendships. We fight alongside each other, like warriors.' But though it sounds cool, it may be harmful, because it forces men to behave in a *certain way* in their friendships, and anything else is considered unnatural or wrong.

It also pushes men into isolation, and it ignores men's need and desire for closeness, one of the most important human qualities. I asked a dude what he wanted the most in a friendship, and his answer was, 'I just want to be genuinely loved and cared for.' That doesn't sound like a shoulder-to-shoulder friendship to me. It sounds like a face-to-face friendship, which I believe we're all created for.

Both men's and women's friendships involve looking *at* each other (face to face) and *ahead and outwards* (shoulder to shoulder). It's not either-or – it's both.

Some also say men are only interested in *doing* things together, and not in simply *being* together. This statement is offensive towards men, to be honest. If a man cannot connect with someone unless he's doing something, he really needs help. Again, a child is fully able to connect and bond without 'doing things' – a child can look at you for ages and be mesmerised by *just being with you*. They're also able to bond through activities. They can do both. So let's not limit men's capacity. Men are fully capable of connecting deeply with other people – some just need to relearn how to do it.

9 A WORLD OBSESSED WITH ROMANTIC LOVE

(A PREVIOUSLY PUBLISHED ARTICLE)

We live in a culture obsessed with romantic love. Finding 'the one' has become the goal of many lives. In most movies, music and media, romantic relationships are valued and pursued at all cost. This culture has affected us more than most of us would like to admit, if we're even aware of it.

'That's cool, but maybe guys just aren't really interested in having these deep friendships, since romantic relationships are so much more valued.'

Well, after interviewing numerous teenage boys about their friendships, Niobe Way says in her book *Deep Secrets* that

> Teenage boys—the same boys who have sex, video games, and sports on their minds and are 'activity' or 'object' oriented—spoke about 'circles of love,' 'spilling your heart out to somebody,' 'sharing deep depth secrets,' and 'feeling lost' without their male best friends.[4]

Clearly, the guys valued their male best friends. But when growing up it's easier to conform to the culture we live in than to go against it.

It's sad to see how friendships are at the mercy of romantic relationships. I've heard lots of stories of guys losing their best friend when a woman has entered the picture. A dating relationship becomes the number one priority in life – and friendships are replaced by a romantic partner. For many men this relationship becomes their only source of closeness and warmth. And as a guy, I sometimes feel it's unreasonable for me to 'expect' a lot from a best friend when he's dating. I just have to settle with our friendship being neglected. But does it really have to be like this?

---

[4] N Way, *Deep Secrets: Boys' Friendships and the Crisis of Connection,* Harvard University Press, Cambridge MA, 2011.

It's good to be aware of the culture we live in and how it affects our behaviour. Let's have a look at friendship in some other cultures:

> Anthropologist Peter Nardi, who has conducted research on friendships among non-American men ... notes the extent to which male friendships are formalised in many countries and provides the example of southern Ghana, where same-sex best friends go through a marriage ceremony similar to that performed for husband and wives. In Cameroon, adults pressure their children to find a best friend, much in the same way that American parents pressure their adult children to find a romantic partner. In China, at least until the late 1990s, and in other Eastern and Middle Eastern countries, heterosexual men, especially those from rural areas, hold hands with their best friends and regularly rely on them for emotional support.[5]

Now imagine doing any of these things in a Western country. People would go nuts!

I'm not trying to say that we should all just start holding hands or have ceremonies for our friendships, but I think it's good for us to get some perspective. Reserving all forms of warmth and closeness for our romantic partner only is a very western way of

---

[5] N Way, *Deep Secrets: Boys' Friendships and the Crisis of Connection*, Harvard University Press, Cambridge MA, 2011.

thinking – and I've been guilty of it myself. However, Niobe Way writes that

> Stephanie Coontz, an historian … blames the decline of social connectedness on our twentieth-century notions of romantic love in marriage where a partner is expected to fulfill all one's emotional and social needs.

She also adds that

> only in the twentieth century (and early twenty-first century), under the influence of Freudianism, have we found ourselves increasingly 'suspicious' of same-sex relationships and focused exclusively on romantic partnerships. These patterns may indeed help to explain the patterns of loss in boys' friendships.[6]

Think about the following claims. I am comparing what's culturally accepted for a romantic partner versus a best friend:

> 1) Moving to another country to live close to your girlfriend is accepted, even honourable.

> But moving to another country to live close to your best friend might be frowned on.

> 2) Being strongly committed to your girlfriend is okay.

---

[6] N Way, *Deep Secrets: Boys' Friendships and the Crisis of Connection*, Harvard University Press, Cambridge MA, 2011.

But being strongly committed to your best friend is a little bit weird, isn't it?

3) Introducing a girlfriend to your family is important.

Introducing your best friend (as your best friend) to the family might make them suspicious.

4) Talking about your girlfriend and how much you miss her is beautiful.

Doing the same about your best friend … Well, it can be misunderstood as gay. So maybe I shouldn't?

5) A movement that encourages great romantic relationships would be amazing.

A movement about male friendships, though … That's a bit extreme, isn't it?

Our culture puts romantic love on a pedestal, which is unhealthy. I'm not saying that romantic love is bad – not at all. It's beautiful. But it's good to grasp the one and not let go of the other.

10 WHAT IS A FRIENDSHIP BUILT ON?

When founding Brothers, I wrote down six values I believe a brotherhood ought to be built on. I did this because a relationship is never built on only one thing, simply because a human being isn't either. For example, though watching a movie with your girlfriend is fun, your relationship will be boring if that's the only thing you do.

Also, every friendship is different, and your friendships can't be identical. All my friendships are different, and that's good. So these values may apply in different degrees to different friendships in different seasons.

Brothers believes in a brotherhood build on authenticity, adventure, loyalty, integrity, purpose and trust.

Authenticity

A man needs brothers who allow him to be real and fully himself, with no need to wear a mask.

Authenticity is key to any relationship. We can't really be known unless we're willing to be open. That means not that we disclose ourselves all at once, but that we don't try to mask who we are, whether with toughness, masculinity or success. We want the real deal! Your friends want to know you, not anyone you're pretending to be.

Several guys have approached me asking how to change their friendships for the better. How do I get past the 'shallow hang-out'?

My answer is this: be the first one to be real – take the initiative. If you want to get to know your brothers more, start opening up. When you're vulnerable, you're extending an invitation to your friend to be vulnerable as well. The reason men's friendships can feel shallow is a lack of *emotional intimacy*. So if you want your friendships to get deep, then you need to start sharing. Share your fears, insecurities and weaknesses – allow yourself to be vulnerable in front of your brother.

Authenticity doesn't mean that you need to talk about how you feel at all times. But it means that you allow yourself to be truly *seen* by another person. Hopefully, the more real you dare to be, the more real your friend will dare to be as well.

Some guys are afraid of being rejected when showing their friends who they really are. But if your friend pushes you away for being honest and showing him who you really are, the friendship isn't strong enough anyway. Second, deep inside, they want to be real. But when you're real, it might scare them. So if you really believe a friendship is worthwhile, and you'd like to invest time and energy in the person, be gracious when facing rejection. If someone has been told their whole life not to be real, sensitive or to need someone, it'll take more than one conversation for them to turn that belief around. It might take months – even years. The question is if you want to give up that much time for your friend. Only you can decide, and there's no right or wrong answer.

Adventure

A man needs brothers who he can enjoy life and all its adventures with.

I am very childlike. I love getting lost in my own imagination. Even though I'm not the biggest daredevil, I love adventure.

The other week I was hanging out with Simon, a new friend of mine. I was visiting him for a few days where he lives in a different city. Honestly, he's the best dude ever. We've only known each other a short time, but we connected straight away. He is extremely caring (when I arrived at his house, he had put a chocolate and a towel on my bed – what a way to welcome someone!), he is super funny, he is very aware of others' emotions (and often reads me and my behaviour), and he initiated some of the deepest conversations I've ever had.

Anyway, one day I went jetskiing with Simon and another guy. Not only did I get to steer it myself, and it got *very* fast, but also we tipped over. We were three boys on the jet-ski, and it tipped. And as it happened, I was thinking, Oh, flip! It's gonna fall on me! I'm gonna die! When we fell off, the engine didn't turn off, so I found myself half a metre away from the engine. I freaked out and swam for my life. I could taste the petrol. Simon pulled out the security cable to stop the beast of a machine – and we all survived … We rolled the thing around and got back on it. I remember we couldn't stop laughing. It was sick. It was adventure.

But though we love adventure, it never comes at the cost of us being caring towards each other.

The point is not that we all should ride jetskis. The point is it's good for a relationship to set out for adventures (whatever they look like). When on adventures, we refresh ourselves and make discoveries. There's nothing better ...

Loyalty

A man needs brothers who are always there, who can support him in good and bad times.

It's easy to be friends with someone when they're doing well, when life's smiling at them. But will you be friends with someone when life hits them and things are challenging?

I've encountered many men who *thought* they had a brother to count on but were left to their own when they were in need and reached out for help. Mutual loyalty, love and support are musts.

We live in a very individualistic culture, and it's crucial for us to *fight* for loyalty in our friendships. And trust me, our loyalty will be tested.

Integrity

A man needs brothers who can challenge him to become a better man, a man who takes responsibility in every sphere of life.

There's a big difference between being childish and being childlike. We're childish when we refuse to take responsibility. We are childlike when we refuse to let go of wonder and amazement. As we grow up, we learn to put away childish behaviour. We're faced with responsibilities that can't be ignored, and we'll get ourselves and others in trouble if we ignore them.

A wise man once said, 'Show me your friends and I'll show you your future.' I couldn't agree more. The people we surround ourselves with affect our behaviour and our choices. If my closest friend treats women with disrespect, that will affect me and my life. If my closest friend starts smoking pot every day, the chance of me doing the same will increase drastically.

Now, let's flip the coin. If I'm refusing to take responsibility for *my* life, that will have a negative effect on the people I care about. What empowers me to change when I realise I've got a character flaw is knowing that addressing it will make a positive difference in the lives of my loved ones – and in all my relationships.

We've all got our issues – and often we're not aware of them. It's only when we're in close relationships with each other that our flaws come to the surface. We're all patient, kind and loving when we're on our own, but as soon as our life intertwines with someone else's, it gets messy. As you develop deeper friendships with the men in your life, you'll experience it yourself. It might get complicated, but it'll be even more beautiful, awesome and adventurous. You'll develop a bond that is strong and solid, build on *intimacy* and *mutual love*.

Remember that we're all flawed, and that a friendship doesn't have to end just because one person's got a character issue – work through it! If you've once said 'bros for life', then prove it. Are you friends for the long haul or just when it's convenient?

Purpose

A man needs brothers who stir him into living a life of purpose, into not settling for less but continuing to grow.

You were created for more than just sleep, eat, work, repeat. You were created to live, not merely survive. In our friendships we've got such an opportunity to build each other up. Honestly, one of the things that has kept me fighting for Brothers and its message is my boys' encouragements. They've told me not to quit. They've told me that they're proud of me and what I do. And nothing means more than hearing the ones I care for the most tell me they're proud of me. I encourage you to pull out your phone and send an encouragement to one of your brothers. You could do it right now.

When was the last time you asked your bro about his dreams? Do you know what his dreams are? How can you help him succeed? And are you willing to sacrifice time and energy to help your bro's dreams and goals come true? I think that's a perfect way of 'testing' a friendship. If we're not willing to sacrifice anything for the other person and for the friendship, we need to either change our priorities or ask ourselves if the friendship is something we'd like to invest in.

Trust

A man needs brothers he can safely pursue a deeper and more meaningful friendship with, without it being sexual or being misunderstood as sexual.

Without trust, a relationship cannot grow, so it's important we trust each other and our motives. We live in a culture that has scared men away from closeness and gentleness in their male friendships, and even in my own life I've often felt shameful if I've been a bit too gentle towards a brother. I've felt like I'm not supposed to be. But hey, I want my boys to freely give and receive emotional support and physical affection whenever they need it – without them feeling weird about it. I also brought this topic up in a friendship once, and yes, it was uncomfortable. But I had to; I knew I had to confront it for our relationship to grow. Closeness (emotional and physical) is important – we were created for it. When growing up, we all needed *female* and *male* love – and I don't believe that our need for both stops as we grow older.

11 AN ORGANISATION ABOUT MEN'S FRIENDSHIPS. SOUNDS A BIT AWKWARD, DOESN'T IT?

(A PREVIOUSLY PUBLISHED ARTICLE)

Brothers' goal is to equip men of all generations to have strong and authentic friendships. We also seek to combat damaging cultural mindsets that may hinder men from having worthwhile friendships in their lives. Though most people love our message, support it and understand why we fight for it, I've heard some funny responses when telling people about Brothers:

- 'What? Friendships between guys?' (followed by an awkward laughter)

- 'Wow, sounds a bit extreme to run an organisation about that.'

- 'Oh, that's interesting … So is it a gay thing?'

- 'A movement about guys' friendships … Well, is that really necessary?'

Little did I know that running Brothers would sometimes feel like walking on eggshells. People have so many perceptions of love, masculinity and male friendships. Post a photo of two guys (a friendship), and some people will think they're gay. Encourage guys to comfort each other when needed, and people think we're trying to turn men into a cuddle club. Write an article about the overemphasis on romantic relationships and how it negatively effects guys' friendships, and some think we're against dating and romantic relationships. And the list goes on … All the stigma and awkwardness around men's friendships is a clear sign that something has gone terribly wrong. And we need to do something about it.

Ask a five-year-old boy about his best friend. He will most likely gladly elaborate about him and his friendship. He will have no problem expressing his love for his friend. Ask a grown man, and his response will be quite different.

Millions of men across the world are facing some pretty serious consequences from the lack of close friendships: divorce, loneliness, addiction, suicide, depression, physical and mental illnesses – just to mention a few … Should we let our culture's prejudice and messed-up perceptions about men's friendships destroy the lives of millions of men, their families and our societies?

With that in mind, I've got one last question to ask in this chapter: an organisation about guys' friendships – does it sound awkward?

Or does it sound like a hell of an important thing to fight for?

12 YOU'RE NOT THE ONLY ONE

When founding Brothers, I started reading books and listening to podcasts about men's friendships, development and masculinity. I did this mostly to make sure Brothers wasn't built only on my personal experience, but also on research and facts. To my enjoyment, I realised that the books and podcasts confirmed Brothers' vision. I wasn't alone, and the thoughts, fears and experiences I'd had in my own friendships weren't unique. They just weren't talked about much.

So I'm privileged to have conversations with lots of different people, especially guys, about their friendships and their lives. Through our programs we've encouraged men to open up and share their experiences with each other. I want men to know that they're not alone. The thoughts they've had are normal, and the fears they have are fears that most men face at some point. And you have no idea how relieved some of the guys feel when I open up to them about my own friendships. They used to feel alone, but not anymore.

I'm only twenty-six years old, but I've experienced lots in my own friendships. I've been blessed by the beginnings of friendships and felt the loss of friendships. I've endured pain, conflict, heartbreak, betrayal, jealousy, comparison, difficulty in developing closeness and intimacy – you name it. I've also relished joy, laughter, closeness, deep love, adventure and good memories. I don't think we can have those first experiences without the others. We can't have intimacy (and I don't mean sexually) in a friendship without self-disclosure – without the risk of being rejected, betrayed or hurt. We simply cannot have love without pain. So whenever I talk to guys who want deeper and stronger friendships, I also ask them if they're willing to pay the price, if they're willing to face some pain as they open up their heart and allow the guys in their lives to really *see* them.

13 MEET AYDEN, MY NEW BEST FRIEND

Four years ago I moved to Australia to study theology and leadership. I bought a ticket and flew from Oslo, Norway, to Sydney, Australia, where I barely knew anyone. It was a big transition. For most of my life I've been quite independent (I moved out of my parents' place when I was sixteen), but living in a new country was a totally fresh experience.

There were lots of parties for new students, and I went to one or two of them. I didn't like them. I missed my home in Norway. I missed my friends.

I remember I called one of my closest buddies from Norway in the middle of the night, crying. As he picked up the phone, I couldn't speak. I started crying even more when hearing his voice. After a little while of me crying and him just listening to me, I was able to speak about what was going on and the fact that I missed him and that I missed home. I knew the move to Australia had been the right one, but I really missed home.

A couple of weeks later I met this really cool dude. His name was Ayden, he was already in his second year at the college I studied at, and he was soon to become my new best friend. (By the way, when using the phrase 'my best friend', even I, as the leader of this movement, cringe a bit.)

Anyway. He was a relaxed guy – just someone I felt comfortable around. One Friday night, after an event, we ended up having a long conversation. It was the first conversation in Australia that I really enjoyed. We shared stories from our lives, and I felt like we really connected.

The next few months, we'd hang out every now and then. A few months down the road, we hung out almost every day. We'd go to the gym together, we'd make dinner together, we'd spend a lot of quality time together. We had suddenly created this connection, this friendship that we both valued.

I remember I once asked him to go out on a 'bro-date' with me. I told him that even though we've known each other for a few months, I didn't really know his *story*, his past. So we ended up having a coffee and some food at a cafe next to the Opera House in Sydney. I still remember that night – first I opened up about my life and my past, and then he opened up about his. It was an important night of our friendship, and I smile every time I look back at it.

Time went by, and Ayden and I connected even more. It was awesome, but I realised that as I was getting closer to this guy, I allowed myself to get hurt by him as well. I allowed myself to 'need him' in a sense. And no, I'm not talking about co-dependency. That's a whole other topic. I'm talking about interdependency, a healthy, necessary way of needing people. You simply can't have deep, intimate friendships with someone without allowing yourself to need them. It's the same with marriage and dating. Anyway, as Ayden and I grew closer, I started realising that I was afraid of being left behind or abandoned. (Yeah, I'm getting personal now – just a heads-up!) Based on my childhood and past, I had created a pattern of belief that people I love will leave me, and there's nothing I can do to stop it. Maybe the fact that I'd been excluded by the boys when I was young worsened this fear.

As our friendship grew stronger, so did my fear and anxiety. In the beginning I didn't really know what it was, so I was confused about why I suddenly felt so afraid when being close to my bro.

Building a friendship with Ayden was the best thing, but it was very scary at the same time. It didn't take long until Ayden noticed my fear and anxiety, and little did he know how these fears would challenge us both.

My wounds were exposed when I allowed Ayden to *see me*, to *know me*. I remember we got into several conflicts – often because I wanted to sabotage the friendship. Instead of being left myself, I wanted to *make* him leave me (by making a scene or acting out). It would make me feel like I had some control over the situation. It was a difficult season for me, and the wounds I had couldn't be ignored anymore. There were moments when I did everything I could to push him away, but he'd still not leave me. I'd tell him I hated him and that he was the biggest arsehole on earth (and I called him worse things than that), but he'd still tell me he loved me. I once punched him in the face as well … Yeah, most people don't believe it. But I did. The story behind it is long, and I'll save it for another time. But the awesome thing is that he texted me the morning after, saying this: 'Well, yesterday was rough. I hope you're OK. Let's meet for a coffee?'

Ayden was very patient with me. He was a real brother, and he was willing to go on this journey of healing with me, even though I'd cost him a lot. I'm forever grateful for that, and I learned a lot about what real friendship looks like because of him.

Ayden and I had lots of fun in our friendship. We both loved adventure. (One of our favourite things to do was hang out on skyscraper rooftops during thunderstorms – we'd both be filled with awe and wonder. One time, lighting struck so powerfully and close to us that Ayden's long hair stood up afterwards.) But I think the depth of our friendship (and the emotional intimacy) was created during the times of hardship and conflict.

Ayden and I were friends for four years, and I considered him my best friend after one year. We've both had our challenges, and we've both had to show the other person our weaknesses. We've been crying together and laughing together. We've made a huge difference in the lives of each other and in the lives of others. I find it funny that numerous people have come up to us and said that they admire our friendship – and that they miss that kind of friendship in their own lives. Most of the time I've smiled and said thank you – because they don't know all the ups and downs we've been through to be able to develop such a strong friendship.

Kim, you're the most sensitive guy I've ever met

I'm a quite affectionate guy. I love expressing and receiving love through physical affection. Give me a hug or sit next to me while watching a movie, and I'll feel more connected than ever. Growing up, though, this became a problem in my friendships with other guys, and in my friendship with Ayden.

Though Ayden was an awesome guy who sacrificed a lot for our friendship, he was new to my way of doing friendship. I valued closeness and affection more than any of his other guy friends – and this challenged him.

I remember he once told me that I was the most sensitive guy he had ever met. I chose to take that as a compliment …

Stuck in the limbo

I touched on this topic earlier on, but I'd like to bring it up here. In my friendship with Ayden, I experienced warmth, gentleness and closeness – and Ayden, though not being used to it, often initiated moments like this. But I also remember all the times Ayden ignored and rejected the same warmth he often would initiate. He could suddenly be very focused on appearing 'manly'. During those times I'd often struggle. I knew he was able and willing to express himself in our friendship, but I just couldn't see it in the moment. Often, as the sensitive guy I am, I'd take it personally. I felt rejected, and I was afraid that I wasn't loved anymore. And even though my head knew that he cared about me, my heart felt like he didn't. Since Ayden could go from hot to cold without any warning, I had to learn not to take it to heart. I had to accept that he's on his own journey – just like I'm on mine. I had to learn to enjoy it when he'd be willing to be vulnerable and open but not freak out when he wouldn't. I'd love to say this journey was an easy one, but it wasn't. I'm still on it.

14 SIDENOTE

A part of me tells me I shouldn't write all this stuff. It makes me too vulnerable. And what if someone misunderstands me or gets the wrong picture of me or what I'm doing? But screw that. I'll write it anyway.

15 COMPARISON AND COMPETITION

Comparison kills

A few years ago Ayden and I went on a summer camp arranged by our church. A dear friend of ours, Kathy, paid for the tickets. She cared about Ayden and me and wanted this weekend to be an investment in our friendship and in our faith. She believed in our friendship at a time when we didn't believe in it ourselves. We had been through a quite a turbulent season, but she fought for us when we were about to give up on each other.

When we arrived at the camp site, it was pouring. We got drenched before we made it to the tent that was set up for us, but it was awesome. Adventure, for sure. After attending the evening service, we wanted to take a shower before going to bed. We grabbed our towels and decided to leave our soaked T-shirts in the tent. It was still raining. On our way to the showers I suddenly started becoming really self-conscious. Ayden is physically bigger than me, and I remember looking at him and thinking that he's better looking than me and he's more ripped than me. Suddenly, I felt worthless and weak. My best friend had become my enemy, a competitor – and I felt defeated. A part of me even wanted to say things to him to tear him down, hoping that would make me feel better about myself. (Remember, this is all going on in my head!)

Then I heard Ayden's voice: 'Kim. Don't do it. Don't compare yourself.'

I was surprised he noticed. But he did, and he didn't want me to waste time on it. I'm grateful he confronted me, because he knew this comparison would be harmful to our friendship, to him and to me. I'd like to say I've never compared myself to Ayden (or other guy friends) after that, but that'd be a lie.

Beware the little foxes

I find it super easy to compare myself to other people, especially other men. Who's the best-looking guy, who gets the most attention from the ladies, who's got the best body, career or house or car … And I don't think

I'm the only one. Our culture is obsessed with these things as well. Be the best, be the coolest, be the hottest, be the strongest. The truth is that there will always be someone better, cooler, hotter or stronger than you. And pursuing these things just brings us down into a pit of depression and self-obsession. I often have thoughts of comparison – and if I'm not aware of these thoughts, and if I blindly feed them, they'll be like little foxes stealing the joy from my friendships. I don't want that.

For me, talking about it helped me deal with comparison in my friendships. It makes you highly vulnerable – but I've simply told my brother that I've compared myself to him, and that I don't want to, because it doesn't make me feel good, and it makes me want to compete with him. And that's not a friendship. When opening up about this, I also allow my friend to see my insecurities – which again will make our friendship more intimate and stronger. And hey, chances are your friend also compares himself to you, and knowing that you tend to do the same can be a tremendous relief to him.

Behind competition hides insecurity

Today I had a really good conversation with my acting agent. He's a sixty-year-old married guy. He asked how I was doing, and I told him I'd started a non-profit, an organisation seeking to strengthen men's friendships, since I'd last seen him. And as soon as I said that, he, with much passion, proclaimed, 'That's amazing, Kim! I'm so sick of us guys always *competing*! I don't want competition, I want brotherhood!' I got so excited and inspired by listening to him talk about the significance of friendship in his life – and he reminded me to write about something important: *competition.*

I've found that comparison and competition go hand in hand. When I find myself comparing myself to another guy, I feel the urge to compete with him as well, and vice versa.

Earlier in my life, I often competed with guys over women. And knowing that I sucked at most sports, I had to make up for it in other ways. I found myself using women as a currency to prove to the guys that I was a man, and it felt even better if it made me look like 'more of a man' than them. Not only is this disrespectful to women, it's also far away from real friendship.

Let's stop wasting time on competing with our brothers – whatever we're competing over – and let's focus on loving each other. You are good enough as you are. You don't need to prove it, especially not to the men in your life you call *friends*. Knowing how bad it makes me feel when I compare myself to others,

I've decided that I'll do everything I can to make it harder for others to compare themselves to me. I want the boys in my life to feel *better* about themselves when they're with me, not the opposite.

16 SEE YOU LATER, BRO

I lived in Australia for three years and then moved back to Norway for a while. Both Ayden and I knew that I was going to leave the country soon, but we both wanted to keep the friendship alive. Maintaining a 'long-distance friendship' takes work, by the way. I've heard too many stories of guys saying they'll be best friends for life but losing touch after a few months. How does that happen? How does it go from a friendship for life to a friendship for a season? I think we often underestimate the power of planning. If you want to keep a friendship alive, especially if you're moving away from each other, a practical plan is a must. And have this conversation *before* you separate. Here are two helpful questions to talk about:

- How do we *practically* keep our friendship alive and growing while far from each other? (For example, should we FaceTime once or twice a week – or more or less often?) Some guys might find this forced or unnatural, but I've seen too many friendships fade away as a result of men trying to 'wing it'.

- Depending on the distance between us, how often would we like to go out of our way to visit one another?

I like to tell guys this: if you really value a friendship, don't take the risk of losing it. Out of sight, out of mind, some say. It's definitely true for me after being away from my brother for a long time.

Ayden and I talked about how we'd invest in the friendship when we'd be on different sides of the world. We came up with some good ideas, and we managed to sustain the connection for a whole year without being in the same country.

I'd like to share with you how I parted with Ayden on my last day in Australia. We met early in the morning for breakfast. I had mixed feelings. A part of me was excited to go, but a part of me was *not keen* on saying goodbye. We ate at a nice cafe, and after that we went to my old flat to pick up my suitcase. Just writing about this makes me relive it all again! Anyway, after we'd picked up my stuff, another friend of mine drove us to the airport. Ayden joined me inside and helped me check in my baggage. Then we went to a coffee shop. He bought us a coffee each, and we sat down in one of the corners. I didn't know what to say. I just felt terrible. I was sitting next to him, shoulder to shoulder. No words were needed for that moment. After a little while he asked if we could pray for each other before leaving. I didn't want to, because I knew I'd start crying like nobody's business. But we did – we prayed for each other and for our friendship. At the end he asked me to do something I almost don't want to share. It's very intimate, very close. It describes our friendship very well. But I'll tell you. He invited me to lean down on his chest (while we were sitting and praying), so that I could listen to his heart. And you might be like, '*What?* That sounds *so* gay!' I'm here to tell you that it wasn't. It was one of the most beautiful moments of my life. I felt connected and loved, and I'm sure he did as well. If you think gentleness and love is 'gay', then you're robbing yourself of the greatest gift life has for you. But it's your choice.

We left the cafe, got to the gate and said goodbye. We hugged for a long time, (I) cried, told each other that we loved each other, and hugged again. We didn't even care what people thought. Nor should we have.

I got to the security check with red eyes. They asked if I was okay, and I responded through tears, 'I just said bye to my best bro.' I wonder what they thought.

17 WHEN THE RUBBER HITS THE ROAD

Many guys come to me saying, 'Me and my bro ... We've got such a deep friendship. We've been friends for years. It's awesome. Just priceless.' But when I ask them to give me a *specific example of this closeness*, they often turn quiet. They're not able to come up with anything.

I've also heard guys say, 'I can always count on him! He'll always be there for me.' It's nice hearing them say this so boldly, but often I find that lots of men *say* they can count on each other but rarely *do*. It's like having a car that you never use – so you never know if it's working.

You can shout from the mountaintop that you've got the closest friendship ever, but if the evidence doesn't back that up, it's simply just a wishful dream.

I moved overseas, back to Norway. Now I know that I'd only be there for eleven months and then move back to Sydney, but I didn't know that then. Staying in touch with Ayden was an effort, but it was worth it.

18 FRIENDS FOR A SEASON OR FRIENDS FOR LIFE?

How do we know if someone's meant to be a friend for life or a friend for a season? I guess there's no easy answer to that – you'll have to figure it out. But most of the time, I think it's a choice. We can't pull the 'friend for a season' excuse when letting a friendship fade. If you want a friendship for more than one season of life, you'll have to fight for it.

I've had lots of friends – most of them have gone; some of them are still in my life. Some are good friends, some are best friends, and some are friends I only catch up with when it's convenient (such as if I'm in the same city as them) but don't necessarily invest lots of time and energy in. We simply don't have enough time to develop and sustain a lot of 'best friends'. I've got to choose between quality or quantity, and I'd rather have one or two best friends than lots of average friends. (As Aristotle said, 'He who has many friends has none.') I'm happy for the friends I've had for a season, and I do think those friendships have served their purpose, but I don't want to go through my whole life with only friends for seasons. I want someone to live life with.

19 DON'T DITCH YOUR BRO FOR A WOMAN

Life is unpredictable. And seasons change. When you choose to commit to a friendship, you also choose to commit to who the person will be in the future (and vice versa). When people change, the relationship changes as well – but that doesn't have to be a bad thing. I'm glad things change. We shouldn't be so afraid of it.

A lot of us want families. We'll end up finding a partner, having kids, getting a house, a full-time job. And all the dads out there will understand that when you have kids, things change. But here's the important thing: your friendships don't have to suffer from this.

I've heard too many guys talk about being betrayed by their supposed best friend who ditched them for a woman. It's sad listening to them when they open up about it. Or what about the guy who gets married and has kids? I've heard countless stories about guys losing their friendships when they start a family.

Why does this happen? And do we really want to just accept (sorry for the bluntness) the *lie* that family and friendship won't work together? I don't. And I don't want to use it as an excuse either.

I believe that if a friendship doesn't survive the various seasons of life, it's because it wasn't strong enough to begin with. That might be difficult to swallow – let me explain: we can't blame our circumstances for our lack of commitment. A child does that – but we are not children anymore. We are men. So if we want a friendship to survive a season, then come up with practical solutions for it go from strength to strength.

If you're a guy and you're about to get married, have you talked to your best friend(s) about the next season? Or do you just want to wing it? You're setting yourself up for a win if you talk about it. How can you make sure your friendship gets the care it needs when you're married? Have a conversation with your wife-to-be as well, and talk with her about your friendships. Explain to her how much your best mate(s) mean to you. If she doesn't understand that, I'd reconsider marrying her, to be honest. I'm not kidding.

By investing in your friendships, you'll also invest in your marriage and family. If you think that isolating yourself with your family is going to benefit your wife and kids or yourself, think again. Stronger friendships contribute to a strong marriage and a stronger family.

Here are a few tips on how to keep your friendships alive and thriving when entering a new season (say, if you're getting married or becoming a dad):

- Do everything you can to facilitate a good connection between your wife-to-be and your bro. The last thing you want is for your best friend and wife to be enemies.
- Set aside specific days for friendship.
- Have an open house. Your wife's closest friends and your closest friends are welcome. Anytime. If your home doesn't feel like home to your best friend, he most likely won't come over.
- Don't reserve closeness and love for your spouse only. Reserve the sex for her, but don't think that she needs to be the only one for you to rely on for emotional and physical closeness.

- If you have children, invite your best friend(s) to be part of your kids' upbringing. You might not be as flexible anymore – but that's all right. Invite your friend to hang out with you *and* your kid(s). He'll become an uncle; how awesome is that?

(Need more ideas? Sit down with your mates and come up with some. Be creative.)

Like with a long-distance friendship, you'll have to come up with practical solutions on how to juggle family, friendship and work. If you integrate your friendships into your family, I believe it'll feel less forced and be beneficial for you all.

To the dads

As a father, you're your kid's greatest role model. If you value friendship, the chance is high that your child does as well. I can't really recall my dad having any close guy friends. He used to work on his car with some of his buddies from time to time, but I never saw him express warmth, love or commitment towards them. He'd mostly spend time by himself or with Mum. I've heard tons of stories of guys my age not being able to recall their dad having deep friendships – and it's a sad reality. I'm not saying this to diss my own dad – he was and is a great dad – but I acknowledge that he isn't perfect either, and he didn't model friendship very well.

And since we're talking about marriage and family

It's no secret that quite a few men tend to struggle with being vulnerable with their girlfriend or spouce - and even his own kids. Quite often, women approach me asking for help on how to get their man to open up and be more vulnerable.

Here's the thing, guys: if we don't practice being open and real in our friendships, we shouldn't be surprised if we struggle with being open and real in our dating relationship or marriage. Us being authentic and emotionally intimate with our brothers will set us up for a win in every other relationship in the future.

20 WHY VETERANS MISS WAR

(A PREVIOUSLY PUBLISHED ARTICLE)

I don't think any civilian has ever missed the war that they were subjected to. I've been covering wars for almost 20 years, and one of the remarkable things for me is how many soldiers find themselves missing it. How is it someone can go through the worst experience imaginable, and come home, back to their home, and their family, their country, and miss the war? … I think what he missed is brotherhood. He missed, in some ways, the opposite of killing. What he missed was connection to the other men he was with.[7]

[7] S Junger, 'Why Veterans Miss War', viewed 13 December 2018, <https://www.ted.com/talks/sebastian_junger_why_veterans_miss_war/transcript?language=en#t-732800>.

A couple of months ago I watched Sebastian Junger's TED talk about why veterans miss war. In his talk, he shares thoughts and insights that I otherwise wouldn't have thought about. The key question he asks is, How can so many veterans possibly miss something as terrible as war? Junger believes they miss *brotherhood*.

Imagine a group of soldiers in combat in a foreign land. They're far away from home, they're far away from safety, and they know their lives are in constant danger. And what they see and experience is nothing less than traumatic.

They know that if they want to survive, they better stay together and help each other. There is no room for selfishness. Their physical bodies and their mental and emotional capacities are tested to the limit, and the nightmare they find themselves in somehow forces them to become closer. What they see is too heavy for them to bear on their own, and they seek closeness and comfort from those they are with.

It's quiet right now, but gunfire and bombs might go off in the next minute. And the only 'security' you have is each other.

In a situation like that you couldn't care less about what's 'manly' and what's not. Leaning on your brother's shoulder would be the most natural thing to do. Pouring out your heart and tears to your brother would feel nothing less than necessary. You somehow realise what really matters and what doesn't.

And then the war is over. You go home to your family. Maybe you have a wife and kids. And you finally get back to your 'normal' life. The scars that the war has given you should make you never want to go back. But still a part of you wants to. You miss the brotherhood.

What is going to 'force' you to get closer to the people in your life when there's no danger around you? Suddenly, you don't 'need' closeness like you used to. Or at least you don't have an excuse to need it.

According to Junger, many veterans end up missing the deep connection they experience during the war. Not having this deep connection anymore is a loss. And with loss comes grieving.

I've never been in a war myself, so I cannot possibly relate to those who have. But I do believe it can be easier to develop a strong brotherhood when in a crisis.

During a war you have to trust others. You have to think about the other and even risk your life to make sure your friend can keep his. But after the war, the ones you've connected so deeply with might be gone or live far away. And your friends who haven't been in the war haven't experienced what you have. So will they ever understand you? Will they reach out to you when you need it? Will you ever be able to feel that strong connection again – knowing that someone's got your back? Knowing that someone would lay their life down for you?

It awakens something in me, writing about this stuff. And honestly, I don't think a brotherhood like that is impossible to obtain outside a war zone. It can be hard to find, but I don't think it's unobtainable.

21 WHEN IT DOESN'T GO AS PLANNED

I'd like to say my friendships are perfect, or that I've always made the right decisions about my friendships, but that wouldn't be true. I've lost friends, and I've discovered new friends. Friendships end for a number of reasons.

Change of season (moving, changing jobs, etc.)

We'll find many guys who'll be in our lives for just a season, and that's fine and good. But let's remember not to use the 'we were just friends for a season' excuse as a cop-out for our lack of commitment or unwillingness to pursue a friendship.

Betrayal

I've found that a lot of men's friendships end as a result of betrayal. And to be honest, I've both *felt* betrayed and betrayed someone *myself*. It is inevitable, but it's important to learn how to deal with it.

There are many reasons why betrayal may happen: greed, pride, desire, conflict, selfishness, jealousy, unawareness – just to mention a few. It might also be a result of a person's poor ability to form and sustain close relationships, which again is probably a result of upbringing and past. The stigma around men's friendships doesn't really help to prevent betrayal either.

What breaks my heart is listening to guys (who normally act very cool, laidback and emotionally stoic) express how they feel let down by their friend(s) and how the trust in their relationship has been broken. My best advice when facing disappointments like this is to always forgive and try to reconcile. Instead of ditching your bro straight away, give him another chance. (You may appreciate another chance too one day.) Too many men just leave their guy friend when they've felt betrayed, without even talking about it. So have a chat with your friend and tell him how you feel. If he recognises his mistake and asks for forgiveness, then good – this experience will hopefully just strengthen your friendship. If he *doesn't* want to own his mistakes, then it's a bit more difficult. You'll have to figure out if you'd like to continue being his friend and forgive and forget without him acknowledging that he hurt you. I can't figure that out for you; it's your decision.

Sometimes *you* might also hurt your friend without being aware of it. If that's the case, then, again: talk about it. Be quick to learn from your mistakes, ask for forgiveness and be sensitive to your brother in the future.

Mutual closure of a friendship

Sometimes you and your friend might just decide to end a friendship. Maybe you're going different ways; maybe there are other reasons you've chosen to end it. I've met guys who've experienced the end of a friendship but never knew why it ended, and it keeps bothering them. Sometimes it's cool to just let a friendship you don't want fade, but sometimes I think it's a good idea to bring a 'closure' to a friendship, especially if it's someone you've been quite close to. You never know if your 'ex-bro' is hurt or confused about why the friendship ended.

Conflict

Often when getting close to people, we'll experience conflict. I think if you've never experienced conflict in your friendships, they're probably not deep enough.

Once a good friend of mine approached me, saying, 'Kim, I feel like we're not getting anything out of our friendship. It's not really encouraging or upbuilding for either of us anymore.'

I still remember how I felt when I heard that – like a stab in the heart. I was ready to say goodbye to the friendship. But what my bro did here was very healthy. He didn't want to end the friendship – he wanted to keep it. And he had observed something that could destroy the intimacy between us, so he chose to expose it. After telling me, we both decided to figure out how we could change. We cared too much about each other to end it. We wanted to fix what needed to be fixed. It's the same with our bodies: when there's something wrong with you physically, you don't give up on your body. You don't lie down to die. You go to the doctor, figure out what the problem is, and then you try to fix it. So when facing conflict in your friendship, fix it rather than move on to the next one. By doing that you'll never grow – and you'll just face the same issues in new friendships.

Different ideas of what the friendship should look like

We were created for relationships with one another. But as men grow up, many are trained away from wanting serious friendships with other guys. Some simply want someone to hang out with every now and then, and that's it.

But if you want a deeper friendship than just a beer at a bar, you won't get it from them. I believe that deep down, these men wouldn't mind close friendships, but many find it too hard to work on, so it's easier to settle for less. Also, we can't sustain a friendship if it's not built on mutual love and support. There is a time to give and a time to receive, and it can't go only one way all the time.

22 BROTHER, I'M COMING BACK!

When writing this book, I told myself I wanted it to be personal, and one of the ways for me to make it personal was to give you insight into one of my friendships – the friendship between Ayden and me. A part of me didn't want to disclose this much about our friendship because I was afraid of what people would think.

I told you about me moving back to Norway (and how Ayden and I had to work on keeping our friendship alive while apart from each other). What I haven't told you about is what happened when I moved back to Australia again.

I missed Ayden a lot while living in Norway, and I really wanted to see him again. One day I called him

and said I was thinking about moving back to Sydney.
I said that I really believed in our friendship, and that I
wanted to live in the same country as him, but not if
he didn't feel the same. I told Ayden I knew this would
be my decision (and responsibility), but I wanted to
know if he'd like me to move back. I told him to pray
about it. A few days later, in the middle of the night,
someone called me multiple times. I saw it was Ayden,
so I answered.

> Ayden: Hey.
>
> Kim: Hey. You know that it's the middle of the
> night in Norway, right?
>
> Ayden: Yeah …
>
> Kim: What's up?
>
> Ayden: I've been thinking. And I think it could be
> cool for you to move back to Sydney … *We're allies.*
>
> Kim: … That's it?
>
> Ayden: Yeah.
>
> Kim: Okay, thank you. I'll go back to sleep now.
> Thanks for letting me know! Good night.
>
> Ayden: Good night.

I ended up buying a flight ticket two days later! The
fact that I'd move back to Australia for a friend felt
groundbreaking – and I couldn't wait. I also knew it
would be good for me to run Brothers from Australia

(partly because English was and is the language of my organisation), and I had other good friends in Australia as well, and a place to live, so I was safe in case anything happened with Ayden and me (knowing that we'd faced turbulence in our friendship before). I wanted to live what I preached. I talk about commitment in friendship, so I wanted to live it. Moving back to Australia was a way of doing that. I knew that living in the same city as my best friend would encourage me and help me to run Brothers. And I wanted to encourage him and help him fulfil his own dreams as well.

Two months later, I was on my way. Ayden knew the day and the time I'd land in Sydney, but he told me he was working that morning, so he might not be able to pick me up at the airport. I was a little bit disappointed that he wouldn't try to swap his shift to meet me, but I didn't want to make him feel bad, so I told him someone else would pick me up and that we could meet later that day.

I'd like to say it was the most awesome reunion ever, and that we've had the best time together since I arrived, but that's not what happened.

A few days before I left Norway, Ayden suddenly stopped responding to my messages. I could feel something was going on, but I told myself I didn't want to assume the worst. He might just be busy, and he'll respond soon.

I still remember the day I landed in Sydney at seven in the morning. I tried to call him as soon as I got my phone working, but he didn't answer. I felt a bit confused, but again I wanted to assume the best. I was going to live with a local family from church, and their son picked me up at the airport. We got home and I unpacked everything. I still didn't hear anything from Ayden, and it worried me. Around four or five that afternoon, he finally replied, asking if I had arrived. I called him and realised that he was at home watching YouTube. Clearly, he had something more important to do than meet a best friend – his 'ally', after eleven months of being apart.

It felt like hell, and the fact that he didn't even care made me feel worse. After calling him a selfish arsehole (and I really meant it), I hung up and cried for hours. Welcome to Australia, Kim! It all felt like a nightmare. Why did I even *think* he'd be there for me? Why did I put my heart on the line like this? Why was I so naive and stupid?

Two months have passed, and after blaming myself for all the issues in our friendship, I started acknowledging that Ayden has some issues with his relationships as well. At one point (a few weeks after I had arrived in Australia) he told me he didn't want to be friends anymore – and a few days later he saw me in church and wanted to sit next to me. I was really confused. Did he want me in his life or not? At one point I told Ayden I wanted to talk to him about everything, but he felt like we didn't need to talk about anything. He was happy to leave this conflict behind.

When people ask me why I moved to Australia, I just tell them I did it because of Brothers. The reality is I did it first and foremost for my best mate, but he backed out when I arrived.

I'm doing good, but it was a rough and unexpected start to my return to Australia. I am forever grateful for the friendship and support I've had from my other close friends in Sydney and overseas. I don't know where I'd be without those boys, honestly. As for my friendship with Ayden, trust has been broken, and even though we had a coffee together a week ago (and everything seemed fine), our friendship had sustained a huge wound that was hard to talk about. And as I said, he felt like we didn't really need to talk about it either. A few days after the coffee and catch-up, he wanted me to join him for another friend's theatre performance. Again, I was confused. I didn't know if he wanted me in his life or not.

I've chatted a few times with another good friend of mine about Ayden and me, and asked him for advice. We both concluded it was a decision I'd have to make myself. So today, after two months in Australia, I called Ayden. After saying hi and a bit of small-talk, he asked me why I called. I told him I missed him and I was confused about his behaviour and intentions. After chatting about our friendship, he ended up saying that he was keen to hang out every now and then, but he wasn't keen on an emotionally close friendship. As soon as he said that, I knew what I had to do. Knowing that we had so much history together, and such a strong emotional bond, I knew I couldn't settle for a casual hang-out every now and then. I wanted a real friendship with a brother who can count on me and vice versa. So I told him to choose: a close friendship or no hang-outs at all. He chose the latter.

Some people have just told me to move on; they don't really get why it hurts – and that's because they simply don't know how deep the friendship between Ayden and me has been. People express so much empathy if a *dating relationship* ends (even if it has just lasted a few months) – but almost no empathy if a *friendship* (that has lasted for years) ends.

You might ask why our friendship ended. Well, that's a complicated question. A part of me wants to write *pages* about what I believe are *his* issues and what *he* 'should fix in his life', but that's not my job, and it wouldn't honour him either. He's on his journey, and his journey is different to mine and to yours. What I can do is reflect on what I've done wrong and what I can improve on and be aware of in my future friendships.

Though a part of me finds it difficult to trust my other guy friends at the moment (because of what happened with Ayden), I won't let the end of my friendship with Ayden influence my other friendships. I need to look ahead, believe for the best and not grow bitter.

I've told you a lot now, and I really find it difficult to share the story about Ayden and I not being mates anymore. But I want to be honest – to show you that real friendship as a guy hasn't been easy, and that you will get hurt on the way. But I believe it's worth it. I've learned so much from my friendship with Ayden, and with him I experienced a whole new depth of friendship.

Important note

Remember that you've read fragments of a whole story, and only *my* side of it. Ayden has his own. He's an awesome dude, and the time we've been friends has been wonderful. I wouldn't be where I am now without him, and I don't regret having him in my life. The guys who get to call him a brother in the future are privileged.

I'm glad to say I had a chat with him about all I've written on our friendship in this book – before I published it. We sat down, had lunch together and went through the book and through the stories. He believed that our story was worth sharing – even the 'not so good parts'. I respect him for that. We're not trying to hide our mistakes – that wouldn't be very helpful to you as a reader either. So thanks, Ayden, for being open to sharing our story.

Some readers might misunderstand or *want to* misunderstand what I've written, but I can't stop people from that. To those of you who are genuinely interested in authentic friendships, and to those of you who've appreciated me being transparent and real – I hope my journey can teach you something. I hope I'm preparing the way for other men to experience the depth of real friendship – and may this let-down set me (and us) up for a win in the future.

23 IT'S NORMAL

Knowing that something is normal, and that you're not the only one experiencing it, is often a relief. But someone has to be the first to share, and that can be scary.

Here are a few things I've experienced in my friendships that I've not dared to admit to anyone else, thinking they're not normal, when they actually are.

Chemistry

I remember when I visited Simon and his family in Brisbane for the first time. (Simon is an Aussie dude I met in Norway six months ago, while he was travelling with one of his mates.) We didn't really know each other, but we really connected the first time we met in Norway. Since I was going to Brisbane to meet someone else, we thought it could be cool to catch up.

I ended up staying with him and his family for four nights. The great thing about Simon and me is that we had such chemistry. I remember he told me that 'it felt like we've known each other for years' – after we'd only been together four days. I couldn't agree more! Simon and I just really connected. We could talk about anything – and we'd laugh together, talk about deep things together, and we simply loved each other's company. I told all my friends about him when I got back to Sydney. It felt like a crush! Like a 'bro-crush' or a 'brush', as I like to call it. He would laugh at all my jokes and make me feel so special and admired. It was awesome.

Experiencing a 'high' or an excitement when meeting a guy you really like is normal, but most of us don't want to admit it. I've felt it! And it's rad; it's like a kick-starter to a new friendship.

'Break-ups'

I've experienced the end of a few friendships, but the one that hurt the most was the end of my bond with Ayden. It really felt like a break-up. Settling with the fact that my best friend is not my best friend anymore is painful, and it takes time – and a lot of grieving. This is a normal and healthy reaction. To me, the break-up of a friendship is no less painful than the break-up of a dating relationship. For some, it can be worse.

Some of you guys have tried to ignore the pain you've faced after the end of a friendship. You've felt like it's wrong for you to feel a strong sense of loss and sadness, especially since it's caused by another guy (and not a woman). I'm here to tell you it's time to acknowledge that loss and those emotions, and don't ever think it's 'gay' or 'girlish' to grieve over the loss of a brother.

Strong emotions

Some guys feel more than others. We're all different. But don't be surprised if you experience strong emotions in your male friendships. For many years, a part of me thought I wasn't supposed to feel deep love for my guy friends, and that deep love was reserved for dating. I don't believe that anymore, and now I'm quick to appreciate these emotions when they appear in my friendships with my boys. Here are some of the emotions I've experienced in my guy friendships: joy, loss, love, anger, sadness, jealousy and admiration. I've also really missed some of my friends when I've been away from them, and the feeling of missing someone has at times been intense.

Confusion

Gotta love the confusion! I remember having an awesome time with Simon for a few days in Brisbane. But when I got back to Sydney, he suddenly wouldn't reply to my text messages. I remember I was like, Why isn't he answering? I thought we had a little bromance going on! I started getting really puzzled about why he wouldn't pick up the phone or get back to me even though he said he would. There could have been many reasons why Simon didn't reply to me – and I'm pretty sure he didn't mean it in a bad way. But how do I get rid of the confusion? I guess there's only one way to figure that out, and that's by talking to him about it. So I guess I should just give him another call.

You piss me off

I've met guys who say they've never experienced conflict in their friendships. I have no clue how they do it, but that's certainly not the case in mine. I've found that my friends – yes, even my best bros – sometimes piss me off. And sometimes I don't even know why! I've discovered that real friendship allows you to be real. Simple as that. When I know that a friend loves me, I'm not afraid (or I'm less afraid) of exposing my flaws to him. If I don't expose them willingly, they'll sooner or later come to the surface.

I need space

In any relationship it's important to respect each other's need for space. Sometimes I just feel like I've had enough of someone – and that doesn't mean I don't love them anymore. It just means I need some space. I need a little quality time with myself or with someone else. But it gets tricky when one friend wants space but another wants 'togetherness'. When that happens, one person has to let go of their need, for the sake of the other. We gotta give and take.

24 PRACTICAL ADVICE

Here are a few practical tips on how to deepen the friendships in your life.

Take the initiative

This is my number one piece of advice for all guys. If you want to take your friendships to a deeper level, take the initiative.

To some guys this might look like being the first one to be vulnerable. Maybe you've struggled with anxiety or loneliness for a long time, but you've never told anyone. Well, maybe now's the time. It won't be easy to open up (most likely), but it'll be vital for your health and for the health of your friendship.

Another tip is to catch up with a friend and actually talk *about* your friendship. Most likely, you've never done that before. But I've found it to be a really

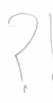

helpful thing. Shout your brother a coffee and start the conversation. Tell him that you value him and the friendship, and that you'd like to invest more into the bond between you. Then ask him what he feels, and if he wants the same.

If you find this really awkward or difficult, you could always introduce him to Brothers first. (You can show him our website or our Instagram as well.) If you have a look at the resources on our platforms together, you'll most likely find something to talk about. You can even give him this book! *Then* you can let him know that you'd like to invest more in the friendship.

Change the scenario

Have you ever seen people change behaviour when they're with different people? I've often seen it. I've often experienced a deep connection with a friend when it's been just us two, but when we've hung out with lots of other guys, I've found it more difficult to connect with him on a deeper level. Sometimes I've even thought, Oh, flip! What happened to us? Where's the connection?

It's natural to change behaviour like that. And it's necessary. It's good to be in groups, and it's good to be alone with someone. But for a friendship to grow deep, we need to spend time alone with each other as well.

A lot of guys hang out with 'the boys' all the time. When hanging out with a lot of guys, I've often felt like it's easier to just go with the flow and not really be as authentic as I'd like to be. Without going further into that, I encourage you to reach out to one of the guys you really like and spend some quality time with *only* him. Go on a trip together. Go for a run and initiate good conversations. Make dinner together one night. Try to find a location that facilitates connection. A noisy bar probably isn't the best place for that.

Start sharing some of your fears, insecurities and weaknesses

Men have approached me, desperately wanting more out of their friendships. They often ask, 'Why do my friendships with other guys feel so empty?' My answer is that they lack emotional intimacy. Without emotional intimacy, your friendships will feel empty. And for your friendship to develop emotional intimacy, you need to be vulnerable. As I touched on earlier, take the risk of sharing your fears, insecurities and weaknesses with your friend. Most likely, he'll feel honoured that you dared to share it with him. But with sharing also comes the risk of rejection. If that happens, try not to take it personally. A lot of guys aren't used to listening to their guy friends be vulnerable, but thanks to you they might relearn how to.

A lot of men don't have anyone they'd consider friends, and if that's you, I want you to know you're not alone. My advice is to ask yourself if there are any guys at your church, sports club, workplace, neighbourhood, whatever, who you'd like to get to know better. If there are, be bold and reach out to him/them. Ask if they'd like to grab a coffee or a beer. Be honest and let them know you'd be keen on getting to know them more. Take baby steps – and sooner than you know, you might have a best buddy.

I want you to also keep a few things in mind...

Building solid friendships take time

There are no shortcuts to a deep friendship. You might have learned a lot of new things by reading this book – and that's awesome. But as you bring what you've learned into your own friendships, don't be shocked if you meet resistance. I've met guys who're

not interested in talking about their friendships at all –
and they couldn't care less about the 'depth' of their
friendships either. I believe those guys are the ones
who need it most, but it doesn't really help to argue
with them. Some guys might love the fact that you
want to invest more in your friendships, some might
not. If your boys don't get this whole Brothers thing,
be patient. You could even buy them this book. By
doing that, you could actually change their lives.

Every friendship is different

This point is very important. We have to approach
every friendship differently, because there are different
people involved. Don't try to fit all your friendships
into the same box; you'll end up suffocating some of
them. They will feel forced and unnatural. Let me give
you an example: the friendship I had with Ayden is
very different to the friendship I have with Simon.
And the friendship I have with Simon is very different
to the friendship I have with another friend of mine,
Matt. We must learn to appreciate the uniqueness of
each friendship, or we'll never be satisfied with any of
them. But the one thing you should expect (or aim
for) in any friendship is *love*. (I know it sounds corny,
but it's true.) A friendship is a place to be genuinely
loved, and to genuinely love someone back, whether

you're friends who meet up every day or once a year. Love must be at the core.

Talk about your expectations

I'd like to talk a little bit about *expectations*. A lot of us don't like that word, but it's important. We've all got expectations of one another, and that's not necessarily a bad thing. Expectations can be unhealthy if you use them as a high bar for your friends to reach and ditch them if they don't. We all need to be gracious and forgiving. None of us are perfect, and we shouldn't expect others to be, but *healthy expectations are important*. And it's vital that, when it's the right time, we share them with each other.

Have you ever looked at a guy as your best bro but then found out he looks at you as 'just another buddy'? It sounds a bit funny, but a situation like that could've been avoided by talking about your expectations of one another. We can't read minds, so it's good to be honest and initiate sincere conversations. Sometimes you'll have different expectations of a friendship than your friend does. If you don't talk about it, and agree on what expectations you'd like to have in common, someone will get hurt.

If we openly talk about our expectations with our friend, we're setting ourselves up for a win. You'll figure out if you're both on the same page – and if you're not, if you *want* to be on the same page.

Also, in any close relationship, relying on each other for support is not needy. I want you to remember that. Too many men think that asking for help makes someone needy, when the ability to ask for help is a necessity in any thriving relationship. If a close friend of mine asks me to be there for him if he's in trouble, I don't see that as needy or demanding. I don't say, 'Dude, don't put that expectation on me!' I see it as a declaration of trust. Some of us guys also put our walls up when someone asks for help, because we don't want to be told what to do. The people we care about should be able to ask us for support without us getting all stubborn.

Know the difference between material dependence and emotional dependence

This is important to keep in mind when developing a friendship, or any kind of relationship. I've talked to men who proudly say they can always depend on their friend. When I ask them to elaborate, they tend to tell me how they depend on their friend for food, money, housing and other material things. But when I ask them about emotional dependence, they often turn quiet. Here's the thing: there's a big difference between *material dependence* and *emotional dependence*. Though there's nothing wrong with getting material help from a friend, don't let that become a substitute for meeting each other's *emotional needs*.

Failure is inevitable

You need to embrace failure. If you're afraid of failure, then stay far away from close friendships. You will fail your friend from time to time, and your friend will fail you from time to time. That's where forgiveness and patience come in. You're not friends because you're perfect; you're friends because you really care about each other. You're living life alongside each other.

Speak up

Communication is underrated. I wonder how many unnecessary conflicts we could have avoided if we'd only *talk* together, and how many friendships could have been saved if we'd fix a problem before it got too big. If you've been hurt in a friendship, talk about it. If you don't feel well treated, talk about it. If you need space, talk about it. If you're really grateful for your bro, share that too.

Don't give up

Finding good friendships isn't as easy as it sounds. At least not for me. But don't give up. And don't give up on a friendship when facing difficulties or conflicts. Work it out. Fight for mutually supportive and loving friendships.

Have fun

Though I've focused a lot on the depth, quality and 'serious parts' of our friendships, it's important that we don't forget to enjoy life and each other's company. Sometimes I just need to go on a road trip with the boys to get my mind off everything else in my life. Sometimes I need to just chill with my bro, crack a joke or whatever. I also love just being quiet with my friends – no need to talk, just be. And I know that if we need to talk, we're able to and willing to. It's awesome.

A good friendship will empower others

Have you ever been hanging out with some people, like a couple or a pair of best friends, and you feel like the odd one out? I have, and I'm sure I've made other people feel like the odd one out at times as well. But I don't want any of my relationships (whether with a friend or a girlfriend) to make other people feel excluded. I appreciate quality time with my bros more than anything, but when we surround ourselves with other people, let's make them feel seen and loved.

If you've got a wife or a family, a healthy friendship ought to empower your relationship with them. And a healthy marriage ought to empower your relationship with your brothers.

Being alone with a friend is vital for you to get to know each other well. But everything in moderation. We don't want to isolate ourselves.

Let it be organic but intentional

There's no a formula to relationships. People are organic and ever changing, and our relationships are no different. Though being intentional and practical is good (and I've talked a lot about that), it will make a relationship unnatural and mechanical if you focus only on that. There's a time for both – to be intentional and to just let it flow its natural course.

25 THE JOURNEY AHEAD

Some days I wake up full of passion, full of hope for the future. And some days I wake up and I just want to give up on this whole Brothers thing.

I remember one night in Norway when I couldn't sleep. I was thinking and thinking about Brothers and all the challenges we've met and will meet. That day I had also experienced another let-down in one of my friendships, which made me want to give up on friendship myself. I used to have a few Brothers posters in my bedroom. That night I got so sick of Brothers and friendships I ripped the posters off the wall, tore them to pieces and wrote on the mirror in my bedroom, 'I give up on friendship.' I couldn't figure out how to sustain a friendship in my own life – it was just so difficult – so how could I lead the way and inspire other men to invest in theirs?

Three days later I was ready to pick up where I left it; I simply couldn't give up.

I'm not a perfect friend. And I have to deal with the results of our culture's perception of masculinity, its sexualisation of love and its neglect of friendship. Everything I've written about in this book has one way or another affected my life and my friendships. Again, I do find friendships quite challenging – especially since there's such a big gap between what I'd *like* them to look like and what they *do* look like. I need to learn to be content with what I've got but still not settle at contentment and continue to strive for more.

Some guys might wonder why most of this book has been about 'deep things' and 'serious stuff'. Like I've said, some might wonder if my goal is to turn guys into a super serious, emotional cuddle club. And here's my answer to that: not at all. The point is that I don't need to remind guys to chill, go on adventures, laugh and all that. Most guys already do that. By publishing this book and by running Brothers I hope to stir the pot and challenge men's mindsets to the point that they want to change them. I want men to step into the *fullness of friendship*, not a dulled-down version of it. And if we as men are uncomfortable or unable to express love towards each other (in whatever form or way we express it), our friendships will never thrive.

So yeah, Brothers is as much a personal journey as it is an organisation, and I believe the journey's just begun. We're reaching thousands of men across the globe already, and I'm so excited for what's ahead of us. I've got tons of dreams for Brothers, and most of them make me freak out (because they're too big!) One of my dreams is to make a movie about a friendship between two guys. I don't think there are many movies like that out there, focusing exclusively on a friendship – and I hope it will rock the boat and give value to male bonding. Another dream I have is to run our programs and campaigns across the world. I believe our message could benefit every part of our society, which is why I'd love to continue to work with companies, organisations, sporting clubs, governments – and anything in between. We want to be the loudest voice worldwide advocating for men's friendships, and by doing that, make a vital positive difference in the lives of millions of men. Anyway, these are some of my dreams for Brothers. And I can't wait to see them come true. It is an exciting journey. And I would be honoured for you to accompany me.

As for your own friendships, don't settle for less. If we allow the culture around us to set the standard for our friendships, we'll miss out on a lot.

Hopefully, this book has informed, challenged and inspired you. My wish is to see your friendships thrive and grow, so that you'll live a better and more wholesome life.

As you take what you've learned in this book into your own friendships, remember that some guys might not be willing to go on this journey with you. And you can't force them to. Every man has to set aside his pride and admit that he's not as 'strong' or 'independent' as he thinks he is – and admit that he needs intimate friendships in his life. But until then, you need to find the guys who are willing to go on the journey.

I hope you've discovered some new things about friendship by reading this book – and you might have also become aware of a few things in your 'friendship life' that you'd like to change.

And as you commit to that journey, know that I'm cheering for you.

Some people ask, 'What about women's friendships?' Well, I am all about women having strong, authentic friendships as well. But I've chosen to focus on men's friendships because men are often exposed to different challenges in their friendships than women.

I can't stress enough the importance of women joining our journey. So far, some of the people most passionate about Brothers are women. That just shows that men's relationships have an effect in the lives of women. So hey, to all the women out there: you have a significant influence on the men in your life. I wonder where some guys would be if they hadn't had a woman 'kicking their butt', stirring them to take initiative.

One last thing. Remember that your story matters. I've often learned more about friendship by listening to guys open up about their own friendships than by reading dense books on the topic. In this book I've tried to share a bit of my story – hoping it'd help someone. You sharing some of your story can help someone as well.

Anyway. That's it. For now.

26 JOIN THE JOURNEY

Brothers is a global movement that seeks to empower and inspire boys and men to create strong, wholesome and authentic friendships and combat damaging cultural influences that can hinder this. We aim to change men's lives and pioneer growth in male friendships.

Join the journey, as we champion men's friendships across the globe!

Ways to connect with Brothers

www.wearebrothers.org

www.instagram.com/**wearebrothersorg**

On our website, you'll find all our resources, information on how to subscribe to our email list, how to volunteer and how support our work – among lots of inspiring stories.

If you want to help more guys find out about Brothers, please consider sharing this book with the people in your sphere of life. Thank you!

Bookings

Would you like to book Kim Evensen for an event? Brothers offers workshops and presentations for schools, sporting clubs, events, companies and other organisations. Send an email to contact@wearebrothers.org. Kim can travel wherever to run a program, so whatever part of the globe you're from, send us an email.

Donate

Do you like what Brothers is about? Do you want to see men throughout the world benefit from the work we do and will do in the future? Financial gifts can help us do that. You can donate to Brothers on our website or by emailing us on contact@wearebrothers.org.

Thank you for believing in our work.

Partner with us

We want to work with organisations and businesses to make a difference in men's lives. If you'd like to partner with us in one way or another, let us know and we'll have a conversation. Send us an email today: contact@wearebrothers.org

Testimonials

We invited Kim Evensen to come and teach our youth group about the core and heart of Brothers.

It really challenged and inspired us to think about our friendships. The workshop Kim had with us, opened our eyes to many things in regards to men's friendships. Honestly, it made us see what we otherwise wouldn't have seen.

—Martin (youth worker)

***

The work Kim and his team are doing through Brothers is remarkable in many ways. Brothers is directly and effectively addressing the many damaging cultural stigmas that prohibit boys and men from forming social connection. Kim's understanding of the issues behind the isolation of boys and men face is ever-expanding because he seeks advice from a wide range of sources and he acts on it.

I have been writing and speaking on men's issues for nearly ten years now. I have seen many different initiatives, which in seeking to address men's challenges bog down in privileged or insensitive frames, thus creating more challenges then they resolve. Brothers does not suffer from these challenges. It is an organization that respects the issues faced by women and people of color even as it works to create much needed connection among men.

—Mark Greene, Senior Editor at the Good Men Project, writer, speaker and advocate on men's issues, founder of Remaking Manhood

***

I found something that I didn't think I needed. And it changed my life. It's so special ... I can't describe it ...

—Julian (Brothers gathering attendee)

***

I used to be in an environment where being tough and emotionally stoic was how you'd behave. I had been taught by society that being open and vulnerable wasn't manly, but being independent at all times was. This affected all my relationships. Brothers taught me to open up, and I've started to express myself more freely, without being afraid of being rejected by the guys. It's a process, but I'm glad it has started. Brothers is helping me to change my mindset, and not let society decide how I ought to behave in my life and in my friendships.

—Jonathan (24)

***

Brothers has challenged the way I see friendship, and taught me how to build real and intimate friendships in my own life.

—Roland (29)
Brothers gathering attendee

Helpful resources

Books:

Deep Secrets by Niobe Way

Breaking the Male Code by Robert Garfield

When Boys Become Boys by Judy Y Chu

Remaking Manhood by Mark Greene

Online resources:

www.wearebrothers.org/blog

www.wearebrothers.org

www.remakingmanhood.com

Movies:

The Mask You Live In (documentary)

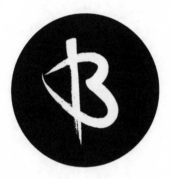

WWW.WEAREBROTHERS.ORG

9 780648 482901